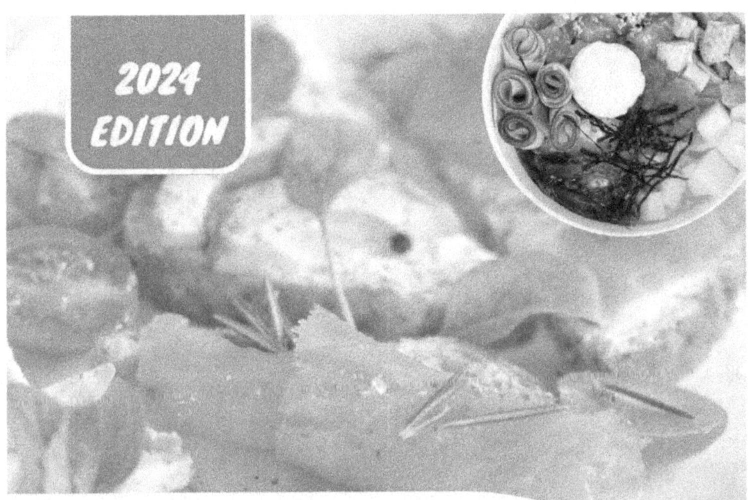

HORMONAL BALANCE
RECIPES FOR WOMEN OVER 40

From Fluctuations to Flourishing, A Woman's Journey to Hormonal Health

Amber K. Padilla

HORMONAL BALANCE RECIPESFOR WOMEN OVER 40

From Fluctuations to Flourishing, A Woman's Journey to Hormonal Health

Amber K. Padilla

Table of Contents

Introduction

Women over the age of 40 go on a transforming journey that transcends chronological time; it is characterized by distinct physiological changes and a shifting hormonal environment. The core of this book, "Hormonal Balance Recipes for Women Over 40," is to recognize and embrace the significant importance of hormonal balance throughout this life stage. In this introduction, we will look at the importance of hormonal balance, the subtle changes that occur inside a woman's body, and the road to managing hormonal wellness via a mindful diet.

The Importance of Hormonal Balance

Hormones are the body's messengers, orchestrating a delicate symphony that affects physical, mental, and emotional well-being. As the body's levels of estrogen, progesterone, and other critical hormones fluctuate, hormonal balance becomes increasingly important for women over 40. These oscillations can take many forms, including changes in mood and energy levels, as well as changes in metabolism and sleep habits. Maintaining hormonal balance is important for more than just body processes; it also has a significant influence on overall life satisfaction.

Understanding the interdependence of hormones and their impact on numerous facets of health is essential. Hormonal imbalances can cause symptoms such as exhaustion, mood changes, weight fluctuations, and sleep disturbances. Recognizing the importance of hormonal balance allows women to empower themselves to control their well-being and optimize their health at this time of life.

Hormonal Changes and Women Over 40

As women hit their forties, they experience a normal and unavoidable change in hormone patterns. The perimenopausal phase, which is characterized by a progressive fall in estrogen levels, frequently begins at this time. This hormonal shift can cause a variety of symptoms, including irregular menstruation periods, hot flashes, and bone density abnormalities. Recognizing these changes is the first step towards educated self-care.

Exploring the complexities of hormonal shifts is not intended to induce fear, but rather to impart knowledge that will enable women to embrace this era with grace and vigor. Understanding the nature of hormonal fluctuations allows women to make more educated decisions about their lifestyle, diet, and overall health, providing the groundwork for a pleasant and vigorous life after 40.

Navigating Hormonal Health Through Nutrition

Among the dynamic hormonal changes, nutrition appears as a formidable ally in the quest for balance. Nourishing the body with the correct foods helps to reduce the impact of hormone changes while also improving general health. This portion of the introduction sets the context for the book's central theme: the transforming power of mindful diet in managing hormonal wellness.

Navigating hormonal health via nutrition entails adopting a comprehensive and sustainable eating style rather than following restrictive diets. Women may positively affect their hormonal balance by making intelligent eating choices, which helps their bodies adapt to change. This introduction provides the basis for a culinary journey that addresses hormonal health while also celebrating the joy of nourishing the body with tasty and purposeful food.

In short, this introduction invites you to recognize the importance of hormonal balance, comprehend the complexities of hormonal fluctuations, and begin on a path of self-discovery and empowerment via a mindful diet. It sets the tone for a book that is more than simply a cookbook, but also a comprehensive guide to appreciating the beauty and strength of women over 40.

Chapter 1

Understanding Hormonal Changes in Women Over 40

As women elegantly enter their forties, they experience a phase distinguished by significant hormonal shifts, a chapter in their life's story in which the body undergoes a subtle alteration. This chapter attempts to decipher the complexity of hormone swings at this time, offering insight into the numerous symptoms and obstacles that may occur. Furthermore, it emphasizes the critical need for a balanced lifestyle, cmphasizing the inextricable relationship between hormonal well-being and nutrition.

An Overview of Hormonal Fluctuations

The forties are a pivotal point in a woman's hormonal journey, generally marked by the commencement of perimenopause. During this period, the ovaries gradually diminish estrogen production, resulting in a range of hormonal swings. Oestrogen, a major hormone in the female reproductive system, governs not just the menstrual cycle but also bone density, heart health, and cognitive function.

As estrogen levels fluctuate, women may suffer irregular menstruation periods, which are a sign of perimenopause. This transition is characterized by natural fluctuation in the length and intensity of menstrual cycles, which indicates a steady loss in reproductive capability. Understanding this overview of hormone variations is critical for women navigating this time, as it provides insight into the physiological changes taking place within their bodies.

Beyond estrogen, other hormones like progesterone and testosterone fluctuate, adding to the complex dance of hormonal balance. These changes are not consistent, and the experience differs by individual. Some women may go through this phase with little disturbance, while others may experience more severe symptoms. Women who understand the wide range of hormonal swings can approach this time with understanding and fortitude.

Common Symptoms and Challenges

Hormonal swings cause a variety of symptoms that, although natural, can disrupt women's everyday lives. It is critical to recognize these symptoms as bodily messages requiring attention and self-care. Common symptoms at this time may include:

1. Irregular Menstrual Cycles: The menstrual cycle is a prominent indicator of hormonal alterations. Understanding these abnormalities is critical for distinguishing between typical changes and potential health risks.

2. Hot Flashes and Night Sweats: Sudden and strong heat feelings, typically accompanied by sweating, might interfere with sleep and everyday activities. Managing these symptoms requires lifestyle changes and, in some situations, medical measures.

3. Mood Swings and Emotional Changes: Hormonal changes can disrupt mood stability, resulting in heightened emotional reactions.

Recognizing and regulating emotional fluctuations is critical to overall well-being.

4. Libido Changes: Hormonal fluctuations might impact sexual desire. Open conversation with partners and healthcare providers can help manage libido difficulties.

5. Changes in Bone Density: Lower estrogen levels can cause changes in bone density, raising the risk of osteoporosis. Adequate calcium intake and weight-bearing workouts are essential for bone health.

Understanding these symptoms not only prepares women for the changes that may occur but also encourages a proactive approach to health management. It is crucial to remember that, while these symptoms are typical, each woman's experience is unique, and speaking with healthcare specialists can give tailored advice.

The Importance of a Balanced Lifestyle

Navigating hormonal shifts entails more than just recognizing symptoms; it requires a comprehensive approach to health. A balanced lifestyle is essential for maintaining hormonal health at this time of life. This section emphasizes the relationship between lifestyle choices, diet, and hormonal balance.

• Regular exercise has emerged as an effective ally in maintaining hormonal balance. Physical activity not only aids in weight management but also improves mood and energy levels. Activities like brisk walking, weight training, or yoga may be adapted to each person's tastes and fitness level.

• Adequate sleep is another important aspect of a healthy lifestyle. Hormonal variations can disturb sleep habits, resulting in weariness and stress. Establishing a consistent sleep schedule and developing a sleep-friendly atmosphere help to enhance overall health.

• Stress management approaches such as meditation, deep breathing exercises, and mindfulness practices are important for hormonal health. Chronic stress can cause hormone imbalances, therefore incorporating stress-reduction measures promotes resilience and emotional balance.

• Nutrition is essential in the search for hormonal balance. A well-balanced diet high in nutrient-dense meals supplies the body with the necessary vitamins and minerals required for hormonal health. Emphasizing whole foods, eating a variety of fruits and vegetables, and staying hydrated all help to improve general health.

In essence, this chapter emphasizes the dynamic interaction between hormonal changes, the problems they may provide, and the proactive role that women may play in promoting hormonal well-being. Women over 40 may achieve self-care, resilience, and vitality by learning the intricacies of hormone swings, recognizing frequent symptoms, and adopting a balanced lifestyle.

Chapter 2

Nutrition and Hormone Balance

In the rich tapestry of women's health, diet appears as a vital thread that weaves its way through the delicate hormonal balance. This chapter dives into the nutritional underpinnings for hormonal health, emphasizing the importance of dietary choices in maintaining bodily balance.

Nutritional Bases for Hormonal Health

The importance of eating in preserving hormonal balance cannot be overstated. Our food choices have a significant impact on hormone synthesis, regulation, and metabolism. Key dietary nutrients are the foundation of hormonal health.

• **Essential Nutrients:** A well-balanced diet guarantees enough consumption of critical nutrients required for hormonal health. Nutrients including omega-3 fatty acids, vitamin D, magnesium, and zinc are essential for hormone synthesis and activity. Fatty fish, nuts, seeds, leafy greens, and fortified dairy products are excellent providers of these nutrients.

• **Macronutrient Balancing:** Hormonal harmony depends on the balance of macronutrients (carbohydrates, proteins, and fats). Whole grain complex carbs give a consistent flow of energy, which helps to maintain stable blood sugar levels and regulate insulin. Adequate protein consumption promotes muscular strength and satiety, while healthy fats aid in hormone production.

• **Phytonutrients and Antioxidants:** The brilliant colors of fruits and vegetables indicate the presence of phytonutrients and antioxidants, both of which provide hormonal health advantages. These substances fight oxidative stress, decrease inflammation, and help the body's natural detoxifying systems.

- **Hydration:** Proper hydration is sometimes disregarded in talks of hormonal balance. Water is necessary for a variety of physiological processes, including hormone delivery and excretion. Staying hydrated promotes normal cellular function and contributes to a balanced hormonal environment.

Women may promote their hormonal health by knowing and applying these nutritional underpinnings to their everyday food choices. This chapter lays the groundwork for the next examination of hormone-friendly substances and practical applications in the form of recipes, allowing women to adopt a holistic approach to health via mindful and nutritious meals.

Essential Nutrients for Women Over 40

As women enter their forties, the importance of vital nutrients becomes increasingly important in maintaining hormonal health. This section discusses the relevance of key nutrients for women over 40 and provides basic dietary suggestions to promote hormonal balance, vitality, and overall well-being.

The Essential Nutrients for Women over 40 includes:

1. Omega-3 Fatty Acids: Omega-3 fatty acids, which are rich in fatty fish such as salmon and mackerel, as well as flaxseeds and walnuts, play an important role in maintaining hormonal health. These important fats help to produce anti-inflammatory chemicals, which aid in the control of hormones including estrogen and progesterone.

2. Vitamin D: sometimes known as the "sunshine vitamin," plays an important role in hormone production and regulation. As women age, maintaining optimal vitamin D levels becomes more critical for bone health and immunological function. Sources include sunshine, fatty fish, and fortified dairy products.

3. Magnesium: This element is a silent hero in the world of hormone homeostasis. Magnesium promotes the action of hormone-producing enzymes and helps to alleviate symptoms of premenstrual syndrome. Dark leafy greens, nuts, seeds, and whole grains are high in magnesium.

4. Zinc: Zinc is an essential vitamin for women over the age of 40 since it helps with immune function and hormonal balance. It is abundant in foods including lean meats, poultry, shellfish, beans, and nuts. Adequate zinc consumption helps in hormone production and function in the body.

General Dietary Guidelines for Hormone Balance

• **Embrace Whole Foods:** A diet high in whole, unprocessed foods is essential for hormonal balance. Whole grains, fresh fruits and vegetables, lean meats, and healthy fats include a wide range of vital nutrients and fiber, which promote general health. Minimizing processed meals and sugar helps to stabilize blood sugar levels, which contributes to hormonal balance.

• **Prioritise Plant-Based Foods:** Plant-based foods, including fruits, vegetables, legumes, and nuts, include a wide range of phytonutrients and antioxidants. These chemicals promote hormonal health by lowering inflammation and oxidative stress.

• **Macronutrient Balance:** Achieving a balance of carbs, proteins, and lipids is critical. Choose complex carbs from whole grains, lean proteins from chicken and fish, and healthy fats from avocados, olive oil, and nuts. This balanced strategy promotes stable blood sugar levels and assists in hormone management.

• **Stay Hydrated:** Hydration is a simple but sometimes forgotten part of hormonal health. Ample water consumption promotes cellular function, detoxification, and general physiological equilibrium.

• **Mindful Eating:** Mindful Eating entails paying attention to hunger and fullness cues, savoring flavors, and developing a good connection with food. This strategy encourages a healthy eating mentality while also encouraging hormonal balance.

Women over 40 can take proactive steps to support their hormonal balance by eating these vital nutrients and following basic dietary guidelines. This dietary foundation is an effective tool for managing the changes that come with this life stage, promoting resilience, vitality, and a holistic approach to well-being.

Chapter 3

Hormone-Friendly Ingredients

Creating a hormone-friendly lifestyle goes beyond individual meals to the kitchen's core foundation pantry. This section delves into the notion of creating a hormone-friendly pantry, highlighting the significance of choosing items that promote hormonal balance and general well-being.

Create a Hormone-Friendly Pantry

A hormone-friendly pantry contains nutrient-dense, natural foods that promote hormonal wellness.

1. Omega-3 Rich Foods: Incorporating fatty fish such as salmon, chia seeds, and flaxseeds into your pantry gives an excellent dose of omega-3 fatty acids. These fats promote the creation of anti-inflammatory chemicals, which help to maintain hormonal equilibrium.

2. Lean Proteins: Including lean protein sources like poultry, tofu, and lentils provides an appropriate quantity of amino acids, which are required for hormone production and control.

3. Colorful Fruits and Vegetables: A variety of colorful fruits and vegetables not only brighten up meals but also provide a range of phytonutrients and antioxidants. These chemicals have protective properties for hormonal health.

4. Whole Grains: Choosing whole grains such as quinoa, brown rice, and oats delivers complex carbs, fiber, and important nutrients that help to maintain blood sugar levels and hormonal balance.

5. Nuts and Seeds: Almonds, walnuts, and pumpkin seeds provide a nutrient-dense crunch while also giving magnesium, zinc, and healthy fats required for hormonal balance.

Building a hormone-friendly pantry creates the framework for creating wholesome meals that actively promote hormonal balance and help women over 40 achieve vibrant health.

Key Ingredients and Benefits

In the search for hormonal balance, several important elements stand out as champions, providing a symphony of nutrients that complement the body's complicated hormonal dance.

1. Chia Seeds:

• **Benefits:** Chia seeds have several health benefits, including omega-3 fatty acids, fiber, and antioxidants. Omega-3s promote anti-inflammatory activities that are essential for hormonal health, whilst fiber assists digestive function and blood sugar balance.

• **Incorporation:** Mix chia seeds into smoothies, sprinkle them over yogurt or salads, or make a nutrient-dense chia pudding for a delicious and hormone-friendly treat.

2. Broccoli:

• **Benefits:** Broccoli, a cruciferous vegetable, has chemicals that help in liver detoxification. This mechanism is essential for hormonal balance because it removes excess hormones from the body.

• **Incorporation:** Steam, roast, or stir-fry broccoli for a flexible and nutrient-dense side dish. Use it in salads, soups, or as a stand-alone vegetable.

3. Salmon:

• **Benefits:** Salmon has high levels of omega-3 fatty acids, which promote hormone production and reduce inflammation. Salmon also has a high concentration of vitamin D, which is necessary for hormonal health.

• **Incorporation:** Grill, bake, or pan-sear salmon for a delicious main meal. Add it to salads, wraps, or sandwiches for a protein-packed and hormone-balancing boost.

4. Avocado:

• **Benefits:** Avocados include healthful lipids that promote hormone synthesis and balance. They also include potassium, which promotes fluid balance and general cellular function.

Incorporation: Avocados may be sliced on toast, added to salads, or mixed into creamy sauces and dressings for a tasty and hormone-friendly boost.

5. Quinoa:

Benefits: Quinoa is a whole grain rich in protein, fiber, and minerals, making it beneficial. Its nutritional composition promotes steady blood sugar levels and overall hormonal balance.

Incorporation: Quinoa may be used as a basis for grain bowls, salads, or side dishes. Its adaptability makes it a great alternative for other grains in a variety of dishes.

6. Flaxseed:

Benefits: Flaxseeds include lignans, a plant component known for its antioxidant qualities. They also include omega-3 fatty acids, which promote hormonal balance and heart health.

Incorporation: Ground flaxseed may be included in smoothies, yogurt, or muesli. They may also be used as an egg substitute in baking dishes, delivering a nutritional boost.

Incorporating Hormone Balancing Foods into Your Diet

Incorporating these hormone-balancing items into your everyday meals may be a fun and rewarding culinary adventure. Begin the day with a breakfast dish including chia seeds, fresh berries, and a sprinkling of flaxseeds. For lunch, try a colorful salad with broccoli, avocado, and grilled salmon drizzled with a flaxseed-infused dressing.

As an afternoon snack, eat a handful of almonds and walnuts for a delicious crunch and necessary nutrients. For dinner, try quinoa with roasted veggies and a side of steamed broccoli. Finish the day with a healthful treat, such as chia seed pudding made with almond milk.

The key to embracing hormone-balancing meals is diversity and inventiveness. Experiment with different recipes, try new combinations and enjoy the experience of supporting hormonal health with a variety of vivid and healthy foods. These crucial

elements, whether in salads, smoothies, main meals, or desserts, serve as the cornerstone of a hormone-friendly diet, helping women over 40 achieve energy and well-being.

Chapter 4

Recipes Section

Breakfast Recipes

1. Berry Chia Seed Pudding:

Ingredients:
• 1/4 cup chia seeds.
• 1 cup almond milk (or your chosen milk)
• half cup mixed berries (strawberries, blueberries, raspberries)
• One spoonful of honey (optional, for sweetness)

Cooking Instructions:
1. Gather ingredients and equipment (bowl or container). Wash and prepare your mixed berries.
2. Combine Chia Seeds with Almond Milk. Mix well in a basin or container. Stir carefully to prevent chia seeds from clumping. Then allow the mixture to settle for a few minutes before stirring again to avoid settling.

3. Add Mixed Berries, Gently incorporate the mixed berries into the chia seed mixture. Ensure the berries are evenly distributed throughout the mixture.

4. Sweeten with honey, If preferred, add honey to the mixture for extra sweetness. Stir until evenly combined.

5. Refrigerate for at least 2 hours or overnight.

6. Before serving, whisk the custard to maintain consistency in texture. If preferred, add more berries and sprinkle with honey.

Prep Time: 13 minutes
Cook Time: a minimum of 2 hours (to allow for refrigeration).

Nutritional information (per serving, excluding honey):
• Calories: around 220 kcal.
• Protein: 7g
• Fat: 12g
• Carbohydrate: 21g
• Fibre: 14g
• Sugars: 5g

Nutritional figures are approximate and may vary depending on the items used. Individual dietary preferences and demands might be considered when making adjustments.

2. Salmon and Avocado Breakfast Wrap:

Ingredients:
• One whole-grain wrap or tortilla.
• 3 ounces smoked salmon.
• 1/2 avocado, sliced
• A handful of fresh spinach leaves.
• Squeeze lemon juice (Optional)
• Salt and pepper to taste.

Cooking Instructions:
1. Gather all ingredients. Wash and slice the avocado. Drizzle lemon juice over the avocado slices (optional).
2. Prepare the Wrap, Place the whole-grain wrap on a level surface. Spread the smoked salmon evenly across the wrap. Place slices of avocado on top of the salmon. Spread a handful of fresh spinach side of the wrap. Add salt and pepper to taste.

3. Fold the wrap around the contents to form a compact breakfast wrap. If preferred, secure the wrap with a toothpick. Serve immediately.

Prep Time: 12 minutes.

Nutritional Information (Per Serving):
• Calories: around 350 kcal.
• Protein: 20g
• Fat: 18g
• Carbohydrate: 25g
• Fibre: 7g
• Sugar: 1g

Note: Nutritional values are estimates and may vary depending on the brands and quantities of items used. Individual dietary preferences and demands might be considered when making adjustments.

3. Quinoa Breakfast Bowl.

Ingredients:

- 1/2 cup cooked quinoa
- 1/2 cup Greek yogurt
- 1/4 cup mixed nuts (almonds and walnuts).
- 1 tablespoon honey
- 1/2 cup mixed berries (blueberries and strawberries)
- 1 teaspoon of chia seeds (optional).

Cooking Instructions:

1. If not previously prepared, cook the quinoa according to the package directions. Gather all remaining ingredients.

2. In a bowl, arrange the cooked quinoa. Top with Greek yogurt. Sprinkle mixed nuts over the yogurt. Drizzle some honey over the nuts and yogurt.

3. Add the berries and chia seeds. Place mixed berries on top of the nuts. Sprinkle chia seeds over the fruit (Optional).

4. Serve immediately to ensure uniform dispersion of ingredients.

Prep Time: 14 minutes.

Cook time: 15 minutes (including quinoa boiling time).

Nutritional Information (Per Serving):
• Calories: around 380 kcal.
• Protein: 15g
• Fat: 18g
• Carbohydrate: 40g
• Fibre: 6g
• Sugars: 18g

Note: Nutritional values are estimates and may vary depending on the brands and quantities of items used. Individual dietary preferences and demands might be considered when making adjustments.

4. Muesli with Flaxseed and Berries:

Ingredients:
• 1/2 cup rolled oats
• 1 cup almond milk (or your favorite milk)
• One tablespoon of ground flaxseed
• half cup mixed berries (blueberries, raspberries, strawberries)
• One spoonful of honey (optional, for sweetness)

• Chopped nuts (such as almonds or walnuts) for topping.

Cooking Instructions:

1. Collect all materials and equipment. Wash and prepare your mixed berries.
2. In a saucepan, mix rolled oats and almond milk. Cook over medium heat, stirring periodically, until the oats are tender and the mixture thickens.
3. Add the flaxseeds and berries. Stir the crushed flaxseeds into the muesli. Add the mixed berries and stir until thoroughly blended.
4. If desired, sprinkle honey over the muesli to add sweetness. Add chopped nuts for texture.
5. Move the muesli into a bowl. Serve hot and enjoy.

Prep Time: 15 minutes.
Cooking Time: 10 minutes.

Nutritional information (per serving, excluding honey):
• Calories: around 300 kcal.
• Protein: 9g
• Fat: 10g
• Carbohydrate: 45g
• Fibre: 8g

• Sugars: 9g

Note: Nutritional values are estimates and may vary depending on the brands and quantities of items used. Individual dietary preferences and demands might be considered when making adjustments.

5.   Vegetable   Omelette   with Broccoli.

Ingredients:
• 3 big eggs.
• 1/2 cup finely chopped broccoli florets
• 1/4 cup sliced tomatoes
• 1/4 cup sliced bell peppers (of any color)
• 1/4 cup crumbled feta cheese
• Salt and pepper to taste
• 1 tablespoon olive oil
• Fresh herbs (optional, for garnish).

Cooking Instructions:
1. Wash and cut broccoli, tomatoes, and bell peppers. Crack the eggs into a bowl and whisk until fully mixed.

2. Heat olive oil in a nonstick pan on medium heat. Add the chopped broccoli, tomatoes, and bell peppers to the skillet. Sauté the veggies until they are soft but lively.

3. Cook the omelette. Pour the beaten eggs onto the sautéed veggies in the skillet. Allow the eggs to set around the edges before carefully lifting them with a spatula to let the uncooked eggs flow below. When the omelet has mostly set, add crumbled feta cheese on one side.

4. Carefully fold the omelet in half, covering one side with feta cheese. Cook for another minute, or until the cheese is slightly melted.

5. Season omelet with salt and pepper as desired. Garnish with fresh herbs if desired. Transfer the omelet to a platter and serve immediately.

Prep Time: 20 minutes.
Cook for 13 minutes.

Nutritional Information (Per Serving):
• Calories: around 320 kcal.
• Protein: 19g
• Fat: 23g
• Carbohydrate: 9g
• Fibre: 3g

• Sugars: 4g

Note: Nutritional values are estimates and may vary depending on the brands and quantities of items used. Individual dietary preferences and demands might be considered when making adjustments.

6. Smoothie bowl with green leafy vegetables.

Ingredients:
• 1 cup spinach leaves
• 1/2 cup kale leaves with stems removed
• 1 frozen banana
• 1/2 cup almond milk (or your chosen milk)
• Half cup Greek yogurt
• One spoonful of chia seeds (optional)

For Toppings:
• Sliced kiwi
• Chopped mango
• Granola
• Coconut flakes.
• A drizzle of honey (optional).

Cooking Instructions:

1. Wash and prepare all fresh veggies. Peel and slice the banana before freezing.
2. In a blender, add spinach, kale, frozen banana, almond milk, Greek yogurt, and chia seeds (optional). Blend until smooth and creamy, adding additional almond milk as required.
3. Take a bowl and pour the smoothie in. Place sliced kiwi, diced mango, granola, and coconut flakes over top.
4. If preferred, sprinkle honey over the toppings to add sweetness. Serve immediately with a spoon.

Prep Time: 20 minutes.
Cook Time: 5 minutes.

Nutritional Information (Per Serving):
• Calories: around 380 kcal.
• Protein: 15g
• Fat: 10g
• Carbohydrate: 65g
• Fibre: 12g
• Sugars: 35g

7. Greek yogurt parfait with almonds and berries.

Ingredients:

• One cup of Greek yogurt.

• 1/4 cup sliced almonds.

• half cup mixed berries (blueberries, raspberries, strawberries)

• 1 tablespoon honey

• 1/4 cup granola (optional for crunch)

Cooking Instructions:

1. Wash and prepare mixed berries. If the almonds have not already been sliced, slice them. Gather all remaining ingredients.

2. In a glass or dish, begin by laying 1/3 cup of Greek yogurt at the bottom.

3. Sprinkle some of the mixed berries over the yogurt. Layer sliced almonds on top of the fruit.

4. Repeat Layer. Layer yogurt, berries, and almonds until all are consumed.

5. Drizzle honey on top of the parfait for sweetness. For added crunch, add a coating of granola.

6. Serve using a large spoon to reach all levels.

• **Prep time: 15 minutes.**

Nutritional information per serving:
• Calories: around 320 kcal.
• Protein: 20g
• Fat: 15g
• Carbohydrate: 30g
• Fibre: 5g
• Sugars: 20g

Note: Nutritional values are estimates and may vary depending on the brands and quantities of items used. Individual dietary preferences and demands might be considered when making adjustments.

8. Whole Grain Pancakes with Blueberries:

Ingredients:

- One cup of whole
- grain pancake mix
- 3/4 cup almond milk (or your chosen milk)
- 1 big egg
- 1 tablespoon of coconut oil (or melted butter)
- One cup of fresh blueberries
- Maple syrup for serving (optional)

Cooking Instructions:

1. Gather necessary ingredients and equipment. Rinse and set the blueberries aside.

2. In a mixing dish, combine whole grain pancake mix, almond milk, egg, and melted coconut oil. Stir the batter until it is smooth and well incorporated.

3. Preheat a griddle or nonstick skillet to medium heat. Pour 1/4 cup batter onto the griddle for every pancake. While the first side cooks, top each pancake with a handful of blueberries. Flip the pancakes once bubbles appear on the surface and the edges begin to harden. Cook and Wait until all sides are golden brown.

4. Stack pancakes on a dish. Add more blueberries and sprinkle with maple syrup if preferred.

Prep Time: 15 minutes.
Cooking Time: 10 minutes

Nutritional information (per serve, excluding syrup):
• Calories: around 250 kcal.
• Protein: 7g
• Fat: 8g
• Carbohydrate: 38g
• Fibre: 6g
• Sugars: 7g

Note: Nutritional values are estimates and may vary depending on the brands and quantities of items used. Individual dietary preferences and demands might be considered when making adjustments.

9. Avocado Toast with Smoked Salmon:

Ingredients:
• 2 pieces of healthy grain bread
• 1 ripe avocado.
• 4 ounces smoked salmon
• 1 lemon for juice
• Salt and pepper to taste
• Fresh dill (Optional for garnish).

Cooking Instructions:

1. Toast whole grain bread. While the bread is browning, peel and pit an avocado. Mash it in a basin with a fork. Slice the lemon and prepare the smoked salmon.

2. Spread the mashed avocado evenly on each slice of toasted bread. Arrange the smoked salmon on top of the avocado. Squeeze lemon juice onto the salmon. Add pepper and salt according to taste. If desired, garnish with freshly chopped dill.

3. Serve for a delicious and nutritious breakfast.

Prep Time: 17 minutes.
Cook for 5 minutes.

Nutritional information (per serving):
• Calories: around 400 kcal.
• Protein: 20g
• Fat: 22g
• Carbohydrate: 30g
• Fibre: 10g
• Sugars: 2g

10. Tofu Scramble with Vegetables

Ingredients:

- 1 crumbled block of firm tofu
- 1 cup chopped bell peppers (a variety of colors)
- 1 cup chopped onions.
- 1 cup chopped spinach leaves
- 2 tablespoons olive oil
- 1 teaspoon turmeric.
- Salt and pepper to taste
- (Optional) Nutritional yeast for more flavor

Cooking Instructions:

1. Press tofu to remove extra water, then crumble. Finely chop the onions and bell peppers. Chop the spinach.

2. Sauté vegetables and tofu. Heat olive oil in a large pan over medium heat. Add the chopped bell peppers and onions. Sauté until soft. Add the crushed tofu to the skillet. To add color, sprinkle turmeric over the tofu. Add salt and pepper, to taste. Cook until the tofu is cooked through and faintly browned.

3. Stir in chopped spinach and simmer for 3 minutes, until wilted. (Optional), sprinkle nutritional yeast over the scramble for flavor.

4. Serve hot tofu scramble with whole grain bread or tortillas.

Prep Time: 23 minutes.
Cook for 15 minutes.

Nutritional Information (Per Serving):
• Calories: around 320 kcal.
• Protein: 20g
• Fat: 23g
• Carbohydrate: 15g
• Fibre: 5g
• Sugars: 4g

Note: Nutritional values are estimates and may vary depending on the brands and quantities of items used. Individual dietary preferences and demands might be considered when making adjustments.

Lunch Recipes

11. Salmon Quinoa Bowls:

Ingredients:
- 2 Salmon fillets
- 1 cup uncooked quinoa
- Two cups of chopped kale
- One cup of broccoli florets
- One lemon
- Two teaspoons of olive oil
- Add salt and pepper to taste
- One spoonful of flaxseeds (optional)

Cooking Instructions:

1. Preheat your oven to 400°F (200°C). Rinse the quinoa with cool water. Season the salmon fillets with salt, pepper, and a splash of olive oil. Chop the kale and broccoli.

2. Cook the quinoa for at least 25 mins or according to the package directions. While the quinoa cooks, bake the salmon in a preheated oven for 15-20 minutes, or until it flakes easily with a fork.

3. Sauté Vegetables for 5 minutes. Warm the olive oil in a pan over medium heat. Sauté the greens and broccoli until tender yet lively. Squeeze lemon juice on the veggies.

4. In serving dishes, combine cooked quinoa, sautéed veggies, and baked salmon. If using flaxseeds, sprinkle them over top.

5. Garnish with more olive oil if desired. Serve warm.

Prep Time: 45 minutes.
Cook Time: 25 minutes.

Nutritional Information (Per Serving):
• Calories: around 550 kcal.
• Protein: 35g
• Fat: 25g
• Carbohydrate: 45g
• Fibre: 7g
• Sugars: 2g

12. Chickpea and Vegetable Stir-Fry:

Ingredients:

• 2 cups cooked chickpeas (canned or ready-cooked)
• One cup of broccoli florets.
• 1 cup snap peas, trimmed
• 1 red bell pepper, thinly sliced
• One finely sliced yellow bell pepper
• One tablespoon of olive oil
• Two tablespoons of ground turmeric
• One teaspoon of ground cumin
• three tablespoons of low-sodium soy sauce
• Add salt and pepper to taste
• Brown rice or quinoa to serve

Cooking Instructions:

1. Rinse and drain canned chickpeas if you plan to use them. Trim and cut the broccoli, snap peas, and bell peppers.

2. Sauté vegetables and chickpeas for 15 minutes. Heat the olive oil in a large pan over medium-high heat. Combine broccoli, snap peas, and bell peppers. Sauté until slightly tender. Cook the chickpeas after adding them to the pan.

3. Season and stir fry. Sprinkle ground turmeric and cumin over the veggies and chickpeas. Pour the soy sauce into the skillet and whisk until well blended. Add salt and pepper to taste.

4. Serve the stir-fry with brown rice or quinoa.

Prep Time: 35 minutes.
Cook Time: 20 minutes.

Nutritional Information (per serving, omitting rice and quinoa):
• Calories: around 350 kcal.
• Protein: 16g
• Fat: 10g
• Carbohydrate: 50g
• Fibre: 14g
• Sugars: 9g

Note: Nutritional numbers are approximate and may vary depending on the brand and quantity of products used. Individual dietary preferences and demands might be considered when making adjustments.

13. Mediterranean Chickpea Salad:

Ingredients:
• Two cans of chickpeas (15 oz each), drained and rinsed
• One cup of cherry tomatoes, halved

- 1 cucumber, diced
- 1/2 red onion, finely chopped
- 1/2 cup crumbled feta cheese.
- 1/4 cup Kalamata olives, pitted and sliced
- 1/4 cup fresh parsley, chopped
- Three tablespoons olive oil.
- Two teaspoons of red wine vinegar.
- one teaspoon dried oregano.
- Add salt and pepper to taste.

Cooking Instructions:

1. Rinse and drain the chickpeas. Halve cherry tomatoes, dice cucumber, cut red onion, crumbled feta cheese, pit, and slice olives, and finely chop fresh parsley.

2. In a large mixing bowl, add chickpeas, cherry tomatoes, cucumber, red onion, feta cheese, olives, and parsley.

3. Prepare the dressing in 2 minutes. In a small bowl, combine the olive oil, red wine vinegar, dried oregano, salt, and pepper.

4. Pour the dressing over the salad. Toss everything together until evenly covered. Place in the refrigerator for at least 30 minutes to allow the flavors to mingle.

5. Serve chilled and garnish with more parsley if preferred.

Prep Time: 29 minutes.

Nutritional Information (Per Serving):
• Calories: around 320 kcal.
• Protein: 12g
• Fat: 14g
• Carbohydrate: 38g
• Fibre: 10g
• Sugars: 7g

14. Turkey and Avocado Wrap:

Ingredients:
• Four healthy grain tortillas or wraps.
• One pound of turkey slices (ideally nitrate-free)
• Two avocados, cut
• Two cups of fresh spinach leaves
• One big, sliced tomato
• Half cup Greek yogurt
• One tablespoon of Dijon mustard.
• Add salt and pepper to taste.

Cooking Instructions:

1. Slice the avocados and tomatoes. In a small bowl, combine the Greek yogurt, Dijon mustard, salt, and pepper to make a spread.

2. Lay out the tortillas on a level surface. Spread a fair quantity of Greek yogurt mixture on each tortilla. Arrange the turkey slices, avocado slices, fresh spinach, and tomato slices.

3. Roll up the wraps and secure the ends. Cut the wrappers in half for easy handling (Optional).

4. Serve immediately, or wrap in foil for a quick lunch.

Prep Time: 24 minutes.

Nutritional Information (Per Serving):
• Calories: around 380 kcal.
• Protein: 30g
• Fat: 15g
• Carbohydrate: 30g
• Fibre: 10g
• Sugars: 4g

Note: Nutritional numbers are approximate and may vary depending on the brand and quantity of products used. Individual dietary preferences and demands might be considered when making adjustments.

15. Sweet potato and lentil curry:

Ingredients:

• 1 cup dried lentils (red or green), washed and drained.

• 2 medium sweet potatoes, peeled and diced

• 1 can (14 oz) chopped tomatoes

• One can (14 ounces) coconut milk

• 1 finely sliced onion.

• 3 garlic cloves, minced

• 1 tablespoon ginger, shredded

• Two teaspoons of curry powder.

• One teaspoon of ground cumin

• One teaspoon of ground coriander.

•1/2 teaspoon turmeric

• Salt and pepper to taste.

• Two teaspoons of olive oil.

• Fresh cilantro as garnish

• Cooked brown rice to serve.

Cooking Instructions:

1. Rinse and drain the lentils. Peel and dice the sweet potatoes. Finely cut the onion; mince the garlic; and grate the ginger.

2. In a big saucepan, heat the olive oil over medium heat. Combine the chopped onions, garlic, and ginger. Sauté till fragrant.

3. Add Spices and Vegetables. Combine curry powder, ground cumin, ground coriander, turmeric, salt, and pepper. Add the cubed sweet potatoes and sauté for a few minutes.

4. Simmer with lentils and tomatoes for 25 minutes. Add in the lentils, chopped tomatoes, and coconut milk. Bring to a boil, then decrease heat, cover, and cook until the lentils and sweet potatoes are cooked.

5. Adjust the seasoning as required. Serve the curry alongside cooked brown rice. Garnish with fresh cilantro.

Prep time: 30 minutes.
Cook Time: 35 minutes.

Nutritional values (per serving, excluding rice):
• Calories: around 380 kcal.
• Protein: 15g
• Fat: 15g
• Carbohydrate: 45g

• Fibre: 15g
• Sugars: 8g

16. Grilled Chicken Salad With Berry Vinaigrette

Ingredients:
For the Salad:
• Two boneless, skinless chicken breasts.
• 6 cups of mixed salad greens (arugula, spinach, and lettuce).
• One cup of mixed berries (strawberries, blueberries, raspberries)
• 1/2 cup crumbled feta cheese.
• 1/4 cup sliced, roasted almonds

For the berry vinaigrette:
•1/2 cup mixed berries
• Two teaspoons of balsamic vinegar.
• One spoonful of honey.
• Three tablespoons olive oil.
• Salt and pepper to taste.

Cooking Instructions:

1. Preheat your grill for the chicken. Wash and wipe dry the chicken breasts. Wash and prepare the salad greens, berries, and other salad components.

2. Season the chicken breasts with salt and pepper. Grill until cooked through, about 6-7 minutes per side. Let the chicken rest for a few minutes before slicing.

3. Prepare the Berry Vinaigrette. In a blender, combine the mixed berries, balsamic vinegar, honey, olive oil, salt, and pepper. Blend until smooth.

4. In a large mixing bowl, combine the salad greens, grilled chicken, mixed berries, crumbled feta, and toasted sliced almonds.

5. Drizzle the berry vinaigrette over the salad. Gently toss until combined. Serve immediately.

Prep time: 42 minutes.
Cook Time: 20 minutes.

Nutritional Information (Per Serving):
- Calories: around 450 kcal.
- Protein: 30g
- Fat: 25g
- Carbohydrate: 30g
- Fibre: 7g
- Sugars: 18g

Note: Nutritional numbers are approximate and may vary depending on the brand and quantity of products used. Individual dietary preferences and demands might be considered when making adjustments.

17. Vegetarian Quinoa Stuffed Bell Peppers

Ingredients:
• 4 big bell peppers, half with seeds removed
• One cup of cooked quinoa
• 1 Can (15 oz) of washed and drained black beans
• One cup of fresh or frozen corn kernels
• One cup of chopped tomatoes
• 1 cup shredded cheese (either cheddar or Mexican blend)
• One teaspoon of cumin.
• One teaspoon of chili powder
• Salt and pepper to taste
• Fresh cilantro as garnish
• Avocado slices to serve (optional)
• Lime wedges to serve

Cooking Instructions:

1. Preheat your oven to 375°F (190°C). Halve the bell peppers, remove the seeds, and set in a baking dish.

2. Cook the quinoa according to the package directions. In a large mixing bowl, combine cooked quinoa, black beans, corn, chopped tomatoes, shredded cheese, cumin, chili powder, salt and pepper.

3. Add the quinoa mixture to half of the bell peppers.

4. Cover the baking dish with foil and cook for 25-30 minutes, or until the peppers are cooked.

5. Garnish with fresh cilantro. Garnishes include avocado slices and lime wedges (Optional).

Prep time: 45 minutes.
Cook Time: 25 minutes.

Nutritional Information (Per Serving):
• Calories: around 320 kcal.
• Protein: 15g
• Fat: 10g
• Carbohydrate: 45g
• Fibre: 12g
• Sugars: 5g

18. Shrimp and Broccoli Stir-Fry:

Ingredients:
- 1 pound of prawns, peeled and deveined
- 3 cups broccoli florets
- One red bell pepper, cut
- One yellow bell pepper, cut
- 3 garlic cloves, minced
- 1 tablespoon ginger, shredded
- three tablespoons of low-sodium soy sauce
- One tablespoon of oyster sauce
- One spoonful of honey
- One tablespoon of sesame oil
- Two teaspoons of vegetable oil
- Sesame seeds as garnish (optional)
- Sliced green onions for garnish (optional)
- Cooked brown rice to serve

Cooking Instructions:

1. Peel and devein the prawns. Cut the broccoli into florets. Slice the red and yellow bell peppers. Mince garlic and grate ginger.

2. Stir-Fry Shrimp with Vegetable. In a wok or big pan, heat the vegetable oil over medium-high heat.

Add the prawns and stir-fry until pink and opaque. Take out of the wok and place aside. Add extra oil to the same wok if necessary. Stir-fry the broccoli, bell peppers, garlic, and ginger until they are crisp and tender.

3. Prepare the sauce. In a small bowl, combine the soy sauce, oyster sauce, honey, and sesame oil.

4. Put the cooked prawns back into the pan. Pour the sauce over the prawns and veggies. Stir-fry for another 2-3 minutes until everything is coated and cooked thoroughly.

5. (Optional) garnishes with sesame seeds and chopped green onions. Serve with cooked brown rice.

Prep time: 35 minutes.
Cook Time: 15 minutes.

Nutritional values (per serving, excluding rice):
• Calories: around 350 kcal.
• Protein: 30g
• Fat: 15g
• Carbohydrate: 20g
• Fibre: 4g
• Sugars: 9g

Note: Nutritional numbers are approximate and may vary depending on the brand and quantity of products used. Individual dietary preferences and demands might be considered when making adjustments.

19. Kale and Chickpea Salad with Tahini Dressing.

Ingredients:

For the Salad:
• One bunch of kale, chopped into bite-sized chunks with the stems removed
• One can (15 oz) of drained and washed chickpeas
• 1 cucumber, diced
• One cup of cherry tomatoes, halved
• 1/2 red onion, thinly sliced
• 1/4 cup fresh parsley, chopped
• 1/4 cup of sunflower seeds (optional)

For Tahini Dressing:
• 1/4 cup tahini.
• Two teaspoons of olive oil
• 2 teaspoons of lemon juice

- 1 clove garlic, minced
- Salt and pepper to taste
- Water (as required for thinning)

Cooking Instructions:

1. Remove the kale stems and shred the leaves into bite-sized pieces. Cut cucumber, half cherry tomatoes, thinly sliced red onion, and finely cut fresh parsley.

2. Make Tahini Dressing. In a bowl, combine the tahini, olive oil, lemon juice, minced garlic, salt, and pepper. Gradually add water until the required consistency is attained.

3. In a large bowl, massage the kale with olive oil to soften its texture.

4. In a large salad bowl, combine kale, chickpeas, cucumber, cherry tomatoes, red onion, and parsley. Coat with tahini dressing and toss to combine.

5. (Optional), Sprinkle sunflower seeds on top. Serve immediately.

Prep time: 32 minutes.

Nutritional Information (Per Serving):
- Calories: around 380 kcal.
- Protein: 15g
- Fat: 25g

- Carbohydrate: 35g
- Fibre: 10g
- Sugars: 7g

20. Quinoa and Vegetable Buddha Bowls:

Ingredients:
- 1 cup uncooked quinoa
- one sweet potato, peeled and diced
- One cup of broccoli florets
- One cup of cherry tomatoes, halved
- 1/2 cucumber, cut
- one avocado, sliced
- 1/4 cup hummus
- Two teaspoons of olive oil
- Salt and pepper to taste
- Sesame seeds as garnish (optional)

Cooking Instructions:
1. Rinse the quinoa under cold water. Peel and dice sweet potatoes. Cut the broccoli into florets. Halve cherry tomatoes, then slice cucumber and avocado.
2. Cook the quinoa according to the package directions. On a separate baking sheet, combine

sweet potatoes, broccoli, olive oil, salt, and pepper. Roast in the oven at 400°F (200°C) for 20-25 minutes, or until tender.

3. In serving bowls, arrange cooked quinoa, roasted sweet potatoes, broccoli, cherry tomatoes, cucumber, and avocado. Place a spoonful of hummus on the side.

4. Garnish with sesame seeds, if preferred. Serve immediately.

Prep Time: 47 minutes.
Cook Time: 25 minutes.

Nutritional Information (Per Serving):
• Calories: around 480 kcal.
• Protein: 14g
• Fat: 24g
• Carbohydrate: 60g
• Fibre: 12g
• Sugars: 7g

Note: Nutritional numbers are approximate and may vary depending on the brand and quantity of products used. Individual dietary preferences and demands might be considered when making adjustments.

Dinner Recipes

21. Salmon and asparagus foil packages:

Ingredients:
- 4 salmon fillets
- One bunch of trimmed asparagus
- One pint of cherry tomatoes, halved
- Four tablespoons olive oil
- 4 garlic cloves, minced
- two tablespoons dry oregano
- Salt and pepper to taste
- Lemon slices as garnish
- Fresh parsley as garnish

Cooking Instructions:
1. Preheat your oven to 400°F (200°C). Cut four huge pieces of aluminum foil.
2. Put a salmon fillet in the center of each foil piece. Distribute the asparagus and cherry tomatoes evenly among the packages. Drizzle each packet with olive oil and season with minced garlic, oregano, salt, and pepper.

3. Fold the foil over the contents and seal the edges to form packages. Place the packets on a baking sheet and bake for 20 minutes, or until the salmon is well-cooked.

4. Carefully open each foil packet. Garnish with lemon slices and fresh parsley. Serve immediately.

Prep Time: 27 minutes.
Cook Time: 20 minutes.

Nutritional Information (Per Serving):
• Calories: around 350 kcal.
• Protein: 35g
• Fat: 20g
• carbs: 10g
• Fibre: 4g
• Sugars: 5g

22. Quinoa Stuffed Acorn Squash:

Ingredients:
• 2 acorn squash, halved, seeds removed
• 1 cup uncooked quinoa
• Two cups of vegetable broth
• 1 can (15 oz) of drained and rinsed black beans

- One cup of chopped kale
- One teaspoon of cumin.
- One teaspoon of chili powder
- Salt and pepper to taste
- Half cup Greek yogurt
- Fresh cilantro as garnish

Cooking Instructions:

1. Preheat your oven to 375°F (190°C). Cut acorn squash in half and scrape out the seeds.

2. Place the squash halves on a baking pan, and cut side down. Roast in a preheated oven for 30 minutes, or until the squash is soft.

3. Rinse the quinoa under cold water. In a saucepan, heat the vegetable broth until it boils. Add the quinoa, decrease the heat, cover, and simmer for 15-20 minutes, or until cooked.

4. In a bowl, combine cooked quinoa, black beans, chopped kale, cumin, chili powder, salt, and pepper.

5. Gently fill each roasted squash half with the quinoa mixture. Return to the oven and bake for an additional 15 minutes.

6. Finish with a dollop of Greek yogurt. Garnish with fresh cilantro. Serve warm.

Prep Time: 87 minutes.

Cook Time: 65 minutes.

Nutritional Information (Per Serving):

• Calories: around 400 kcal.

• Protein: 17g

• Fat: 5g

• Carbohydrate: 80g

• Fibre: 15g

• Sugars: 4g

Note: Nutritional numbers arc approximate and may vary depending on the brand and quantity of products used. Individual dietary preferences and demands might be considered when making adjustments.

23. Mushroom and Spinach Chickpea Pasta:

Ingredients:

• 8 ounces chickpea pasta

• One tablespoon of olive oil

• Two cups of cut cremini mushrooms

• 3 garlic cloves, minced

• Four cups of fresh spinach

• One can (15 oz) of drained and washed chickpeas

* One teaspoon of dried Italian herbs.
* Salt and pepper to taste.
* 1/4 cup shredded Parmesan cheese (optional)
* Red pepper flakes as garnish (optional)

Cooking Instructions:

1. Cook the chickpea pasta per the package directions. Slice cremini mushrooms, slice garlic, and drain and rinse the chickpeas.

2. In a large pan, heat the olive oil over medium heat. Combine the cut mushrooms and minced garlic. Sauté mushrooms until they are soft.

3. Add the fresh spinach and chickpeas to the skillet. Cook until the spinach has wilted and the chickpeas are cooked through.

4. Drain the cooked pasta and transfer it to the skillet. Toss everything together.

5. Season with dried Italian herbs, salt, and pepper. Optionally, top with grated Parmesan and red pepper flakes. Serve immediately.

Prep time: 29 minutes.
Cook Time: 15 minutes.

Nutritional Information (Per Serving):
* Calories: around 400 kcal.

- Protein: 20g
- Fat: 8g
- Carbohydrate: 65g
- Fibre: 15g
- Sugars: 4g

24. Grilled Turkey Burgers with Sweet Potato Wedges:

Ingredients:

For the Turkey Hamburgers:
- One pound of lean ground turkey
- 1/2 cup breadcrumbs, whole wheat or gluten-free.
- 1 egg
- One teaspoon of garlic powder.
- One teaspoon of onion powder.
- Add salt and pepper to taste.
- Whole-grain hamburger buns
- Toppings: lettuce, tomatoes, and avocado

For the Sweet Potato Wedges:
- Cut 2 big sweet potatoes into wedges.
- Two teaspoons of olive oil.
- One teaspoon of paprika.

- One teaspoon of garlic powder.
- Add salt and pepper to taste.

Cooking Instructions:

1. Pre-heat the grill or grill pan. Set the oven to 425°F (220°C) for the sweet potato wedges.

2. In a mixing dish, combine ground turkey, breadcrumbs, egg, garlic powder, onion powder, salt, and pepper. Shape the mixture into hamburger patties.

3. Grill the turkey burgers for 5-6 minutes per side, or until well cooked.

4. Combine the olive oil, salt, pepper, paprika, and garlic powder with the sweet potato wedges. Spread them out on a baking sheet and roast them in a preheated oven for 15-20 minutes, until golden and crispy.

5. Burgers can be assembled in 5 minutes. Toast whole-grain hamburger buns. Put together burgers with grilled turkey patties, lettuce, tomato, and avocado slices.

6. Serve the turkey burgers with sweet potato wedges.

Prep Time: 52 minutes.
Cook Time: 32 minutes.

Nutritional Information (per portion, omitting the bun):
• Calories: around 350 kcal.
• Protein: 30g
• Fat: 15g
• Carbohydrate: 30g
• Fibre: 5g
• Sugars: 4g

Note: Nutritional numbers are approximate and may vary depending on the brand and quantity of products used. Individual dietary preferences and demands might be considered when making adjustments.

25. Cauliflower and Chickpea Curry:

Ingredients:
• 1 cauliflower, chopped into florets
• One can (15 oz) of drained and washed chickpeas
• 1 finely sliced onion
• 3 garlic cloves, minced
• 1 tablespoon ginger, shredded
• One can (14 ounces) of chopped tomatoes

- One can (14 ounces) coconut milk
- Two teaspoons of curry powder.
- One teaspoon of ground cumin
- One teaspoon of ground coriander.
- 1/2 teaspoon turmeric
- One tablespoon of olive oil.
- Salt and pepper to taste.
- Fresh cilantro as garnish
- Cooked brown rice to serve.

Cooking instructions:

1. Cut the cauliflower into florets. Finely cut the onion; mince the garlic; and grate the ginger.

2. In a big saucepan, heat the olive oil over medium heat. Combine the chopped onions, garlic, and ginger. Sauté till fragrant.

3. Combine curry powder, ground cumin, ground coriander, turmeric, salt, and pepper. Add cauliflower florets and chickpeas. Sauté for several minutes.

4. Simmer with tomatoes and coconut milk for 25 minutes. Pour in the chopped tomatoes and coconut milk. Bring to a boil, then reduce the heat, cover, and cook until the cauliflower is soft.

5. Adjust the seasoning as required. Serve the curry alongside cooked brown rice. Garnish with fresh cilantro.

Prep Time: 32 minutes.
Cook Time: 35 minutes.

Nutritional values (per serving, excluding rice):
• Calories: around 350 kcal.
• Protein: 12g
• Fat: 20g
• Carbohydrate: 35g
• Fibre: 10g
• Sugars: 8g

26. Lemon Garlic Herb Chicken and Roasted Vegetables

Ingredients:

For Chicken:
• Four boneless and skinless chicken breasts
• Two teaspoons of olive oil
• 3 garlic cloves, minced
• 1 tablespoon of fresh lemon juice

- One teaspoon of dried thyme
- 1 teaspoon dried rosemary
- Salt and pepper to taste

For the Roasted Vegetables:

- 4 cups mixed veggies (chopped carrots, bell peppers, and zucchini)
- One tablespoon of olive oil.
- Salt and pepper to taste.

Cooking Instructions:

1. Preheat your oven to 400°F (200°C). Place the chicken breasts in a bowl.

2. In a small bowl, combine olive oil, minced garlic, lemon juice, thyme, rosemary, salt, and pepper. Pour the marinade over the chicken breasts and leave to marinate for at least 10 minutes.

3. Chop the mixed veggies into bite-size pieces. Toss them in olive oil, salt, and pepper.

4. Arrange the marinated chicken breasts on one side of a baking sheet. Arrange the mixed veggies on the other side. Roast in a preheated oven for about 25 minutes, or until the chicken is fully cooked and the veggies are soft.

5. Let the chicken rest for a few minutes before slicing. Serve the sliced chicken alongside roasted veggies.

Prep Time: 45 minutes.
Cook Time: 25 minutes.

Nutritional Information (Per Serving):
• Calories: around 320 kcal.
• Protein: 30g
• Fat: 15g
• Carbohydrate: 15g
• Fibre: 5g
• Sugars: 6g

Note: Nutritional numbers are approximate and may vary depending on the brand and quantity of products used. Individual dietary preferences and demands might be considered when making adjustments.

27. Vegetarian Lentil and Sweet Potato Stew:

Ingredients:

- 1 cup dried green or brown lentils, washed
- two sweet potatoes, peeled and chopped
- 1 finely sliced onion.
- 3 garlic cloves, minced
- One can (14 ounces) of chopped tomatoes
- Four cups of veggie broth.
- One teaspoon of ground cumin
- One teaspoon of smoked paprika.
- 1/2 teaspoon ground coriander.
- Add salt and pepper to taste.
- Two cups of chopped kale.
- One tablespoon of olive oil.
- Fresh parsley as garnish
- Greek yogurt to serve (optional)

Cooking Instructions:

1. Rinse the lentils in cold water. Peel and dice the sweet potatoes. Finely cut the onion, then mince the garlic.

2. In a big saucepan, heat the olive oil over medium heat. Add the chopped onion and garlic. Sauté until soft.

3. Stir in the lentils and cubed sweet potatoes. Combine the ground cumin, smoked paprika, ground coriander, salt, and pepper.

4. Add in the diced tomatoes and veggie broth. Bring to a boil, then decrease heat, cover, and cook for 30 minutes, or until lentils and sweet potatoes are cooked.

5. Stir in the chopped kale and simmer until wilted. Adjust seasoning as required. Garnish with fresh parsley. Add a dollop of Greek yogurt if preferred.

Prep Time is 60 minutes.
Cooking Time: 40 minutes.

Nutritional Information (Per Serving):
• Calories: around 300 kcal.
• Protein: 15g
• Fat: 3g
• Carbohydrate: 55g.
• Fibre: 15g
• Sugars: 8g

28. Shrimp and Avocado Salad:

Ingredients:
• 1 pound big prawns, peeled and deveined
• 2 avocados, diced
• One cup of cherry tomatoes, halved

- 1 cucumber, diced
- 1/4 cup finely chopped red onion
- 1/4 cup fresh cilantro, chopped
- Juice from two limes
- Two teaspoons of olive oil
- Add salt and pepper to taste
- Mixed greens to serve

Cooking Instructions:

1. Peel and devein the prawns. Chop avocados, cherry tomatoes, cucumber, and red onion. Chop the fresh cilantro.

2. In a skillet, heat the olive oil over medium-high. Cook the prawns for 2-3 minutes per side, until pink and opaque.

3. In a large mixing dish, add cooked prawns, diced avocado, cherry tomatoes, cucumber, red onion, and chopped cilantro.

4. Drizzle lime juice over the salad. Combine the olive oil, salt, and pepper. Toss to coat.

5. Serve the prawn and avocado salad on a bed of mixed greens.

Prep time: 34 minutes.
Cook Time: 5 minutes.

Nutritional Information (Per Serving):
• Calories: around 350 kcal.
• Protein: 25g
• Fat: 20g
• Carbohydrate: 20g
• Fibre: 10g
• Sugars: 4g

Note: Nutritional numbers are approximate and may vary depending on the brand and quantity of products used. Individual dietary preferences and demands might be considered when making adjustments.

29. Eggplant and Chickpea Stir-Fry:

Ingredients:
• one big aubergine, cubed
• One can (15 oz) of drained and washed chickpeas
• One red bell pepper, cut
• One yellow bell pepper, cut
• One finely sliced onion
• 3 garlic cloves, minced
• Two teaspoons of soy sauce
• One tablespoon of hoisin sauce

- One tablespoon of rice vinegar
- One tablespoon of sesame oil
- 1 teaspoon grated ginger
- Two teaspoons of olive oil
- Sesame seeds as garnish
- Green onions as garnish
- Cooked brown rice to serve

Cooking Instructions:

1. Cube the eggplant, slice the bell peppers and finely slice the onion. Drain and rinse the chickpeas. Mince garlic and grate ginger.

2. In a large wok or pan, heat olive oil over medium-high heat. Combine the chopped onion, bell peppers, and cubed eggplant. Stir sauté until the veggies are soft.

3. Add the drained chickpeas to the wok. In a small bowl, combine the soy sauce, hoisin sauce, rice vinegar, sesame oil, and grated ginger. Pour the sauce over the veggies and chickpeas.

4. Stir-fry everything until evenly coated and cooked through. Serve the aubergine and chickpea stir•fry with cooked brown rice. Add chopped green onions and sesame seeds as garnish.

Prep time: 40 minutes.

• **Cook Time: 20 minutes.**

Nutritional values (per serving, excluding rice):
• Calories: around 320 kcal.
• Protein: 10g
• Fat: 15g
• Carbohydrate: 40g
• Fibre: 12g
• Sugars: 12g

30. Turkey and Quinoa Stuffed Peppers:

Ingredients:
• 4 big bell peppers, half with seeds removed
• One pound of lean ground turkey
• One cup of cooked quinoa
• 1 Can (15 oz) of drained and rinsed black beans
• 1 cup fresh or frozen corn kernel
• One cup of chopped tomatoes
• One teaspoon of cumin
• One teaspoon of chili powder
• Salt and pepper to taste
• 1 cup shredded cheese (either cheddar or Mexican blend)

• Fresh cilantro as garnish
• Greek yogurt or salsa to serve (optional)

Cooking Instructions:

1. Preheat your oven to 375°F (190°C). Cut bell peppers in half and remove seeds.

2. Cook the ground turkey in a pan until browned. In a large mixing bowl, combine the cooked turkey, quinoa, black beans, corn, chopped tomatoes, cumin, chili powder, salt and pepper.

3. Fill each bell pepper half with the turkey-quinoa mixture. Put the stuffed peppers in a baking tray.

4. Sprinkle shredded cheese over each filled pepper. Bake in a preheated oven for approximately 25 minutes, or until the peppers are soft.

5. Garnish with fresh cilantro. Top with a dollop of Greek yogurt or salsa if preferred.

Prep time: 45 minutes.
Cooking Time: 40 minutes.

Nutritional Information (Per Serving):
• Calories: around 380 kcal.
• Protein: 28g
• Fat: 15g
• Carbohydrate: 35g

• Fibre: 8g
• Sugars: 7g

Note: Nutritional numbers are approximate and may vary depending on the brand and quantity of products used. Individual dietary preferences and demands might be considered when making adjustments.

Snack Recipes

31. Greek Yoghurt Parfait.

Ingredients:
- 1 cup Greek yogurt
- 1/2 cup mixed berries (blueberries, strawberries, raspberries)
- 2 tablespoons granola
- 1 tablespoon honey

Instructions:
1. In a glass or dish, place half of the Greek yogurt.
2. Place half of the mixed berries on top of the yogurt.
3. Add one spoonful of granola to the berries.
4. Drizzle in half of the honey.
5. Repeat layering with the remaining ingredients.
6. Serve immediately and enjoy!

Prep time: 5 minutes.
Nutritional Information (Approximate):
- Calories: 300 kcal.
- Protein: 20g

- Fat: 8g
- Carbohydrate: 40g
- Fibre: 6g
- Sugars: 24g

32. Trail Mix of Nuts and Seeds

Ingredients:
- 1/2 cup almonds
- 1/4 cup walnuts.
- Two teaspoons of pumpkin seeds
- Two teaspoons of sunflower seeds
- 1/4 cup dried cranberries

Instructions:
1. In a mixing dish, blend almonds, walnuts, pumpkin seeds, sunflower seeds, and dried cranberries.
2. Mix well to achieve equitable distribution of components.
3. Keep in an airtight container for a fast and healthy snack.

Prep time: 5 minutes.
Nutritional Information (Approximate):

- Calories: 350 kcal.
- Protein: 10g
- Fat: 28g
- Carbohydrate: 20g
- Fibre: 5g
- Sugars: 10g

33. Hummus and Vegetable Sticks:

Ingredients:

- 1 cup hummus, store-bought or homemade.
- One cup of carrot sticks.
- One cup of cucumber slices.
- 1 cup bell pepper slices, varied colors

Instructions:

1. Place carrot sticks, cucumber slices, and bell pepper strips on a serving platter.
2. Put the hummus in a dish in the center of the platter.
3. Dip the vegetable sticks in the hummus and enjoy!

Prep time: 10 minutes.
Nutritional Information (Approximate):

- Calories: 250 kcal.
- Protein: 10g
- Fat: 15g
- Carbohydrate: 25g
- Fibre: 10g
- Sugars: 5g

34. Chia Seed Pudding.

Ingredients:
- 1/4 cup chia seeds
- 1 cup almond milk (or your chosen milk)
- 1/2 teaspoon vanilla extract
- 1 tablespoon maple syrup, and mixed berries for topping.

Instructions:
1. In a dish, combine the chia seeds, almond milk, vanilla extract, and maple syrup.
2. Stir thoroughly and refrigerate for at least 2 hours or overnight.
3. Before serving, whisk the custard again to achieve a smooth texture.
4. Garnish with mixed berries or your favorite fruit.
5. Enjoy the chia seed pudding!

Prep time: 5 minutes (plus chilling time)
Nutritional Information (Approximate):
• Calories: 200 kcal.
• Protein: 6g
• Fat: 10g
• Carbohydrate: 20g
• Fibre: 10g
• Sugars: 8g

35. Nut Butter Apple Slices:

Ingredients:
• 1 apple, cut
• Two tablespoons of almond or peanut butter.
• Optional toppings include chia seeds or crumbled nuts.

Instructions:
1. Cut apples into thin rounds.
2. Spread almond or peanut butter on each apple slice.
3. If preferred, add chia seeds or smashed nuts on the top.
4. Place on a dish and serve immediately.

Prep time: 5 minutes.
Nutritional Information (Approximate):
• Calories: 180 kcal.

• Protein: 4g

• Fat: 12g

• carbs: 18g

• Fibre: 5g

• Sugars: 12g

36. Roasted Chickpeas.

Ingredients:
• 1 can (15 oz) of drained and rinsed chickpeas
• 1 tablespoon olive oil
• 1 teaspoon cumin
• 1 teaspoon paprika
• Add salt to taste.

Instructions:
1. Preheat oven to 400°F (200°C).
2. Dry the chickpeas with a paper towel.
3. In a bowl, combine the chickpeas, olive oil, cumin, paprika, and salt.

4. Arrange the chickpeas on a baking sheet in a single layer.

5. Roast for 25-30 minutes, shaking the pan halfway through to ensure uniform cooking.

6. Once crispy, remove from the oven and allow to cool.

7. Serve as a crispy snack.

Prep Time: 5 minutes (plus baking time).
Cooking Time: 25-30 minutes.

Nutritional Information (Approximate):
• Calories: 200 kcal.
• Protein: 8g
• Fat: 7g
• Carbohydrate: 28g
• Fibre: 8g
• Sugars: 5g

37. Cottage Cheese with Pineapple:

Ingredients:
• 1 cup cottage cheese
• 1 cup fresh pineapple pieces

Instructions:

1. Scoop cottage cheese into a bowl.

2. Garnish with fresh pineapple pieces.

3. Gently mix everything.

4. Serve immediately.

Prep time: 5 minutes.

Nutritional Information (Approximate):

• Calories: 250 kcal.

• Protein: 28g

• Fat: 8g

• Carbohydrate: 20g

• Fibre: 2g

• Sugars: 15g

38. Seaweed Snacks:

Ingredients:

•1 bag of roasted seaweed sheets.

Instructions:

1. Open the pack of roasted seaweed sheets.

2. If desired, break them into smaller pieces.

3. Savour these nutrient-dense seaweed nibbles on your own.

Prep time: 2 minutes.

Nutritional Information (Approximate):

• Calories: 30 kcal.

• Protein: 2g

• Fat: 2g

• carbs: 1g

• Fibre: 1g.

39. Turmeric Roasted Nuts.

Ingredients:

• 1 cup mixed nuts (almonds, walnuts, cashews)

• 1 tablespoon olive oil

• 1 teaspoon powdered turmeric

• 1/2 teaspoon cayenne pepper

• 1 tablespoon maple syrup (optional)

• Add salt to taste.

Instructions:

1. Preheat the oven to 350°F/175°C.

2. In a bowl, combine the nuts, olive oil, powdered turmeric, cayenne pepper, and optional maple syrup.

3. Place the nut mixture on a baking sheet in a single layer.

4. Roast in the oven for 10-15 minutes, stirring halfway.

5. Remove from the oven after the nuts are toasted and aromatic.

6. Season with salt and let cool before serving.

Prep time: 5 minutes.
Cooking Time: 10-15 minutes.

Nutritional Information (Approximate):
• Calories: 200 kcal.
• Protein: 6g
• Fat: 17g
• Carbohydrate: 8g
• Fibre: 3g
• Sugars: 2g

40. Yoghurt & Berry Smoothie:

Ingredients:
•1 cup Greek yogurt
• half cup mixed berries (strawberries, blueberries, raspberries)
• 1/2 frozen banana
• One spoonful of chia seeds

• 1/2 cup almond milk
• Ice cubes (Optional)

Instructions:

1. In a blender, mix Greek yogurt, mixed berries, frozen banana, chia seeds, and almond milk.
2. Blend until smooth.
3. If you want a cooler consistency, add ice cubes and mix again.
4. Pour into a glass and enjoy this refreshing and nutrient-dense smoothie.

Prep time: 5 minutes.

Nutritional Information (Approximate):
• Calories: 250 kcal.
Protein: 15g, fat: 10g.
• Carbohydrate: 30g
• Fibre: 8g
• Sugars: 18g

Dessert Recipes

41. Dark Chocolate and Berry Parfait:

Ingredients:
• 1 cup Greek yogurt.
• 1/2 cup mixed berries (blueberries, strawberries, raspberries)
• 2 tablespoons dark chocolate chips or grated dark chocolate.
• One tablespoon of honey or maple syrup (optional)

Instructions:
1. In a glass or dish, place half of the Greek yogurt.
2. Place half of the mixed berries on top of the yogurt.
3. Add one tablespoon of dark chocolate chips or shredded dark chocolate.
4. Optionally, drizzle with half of the honey or maple syrup.
5. Repeat layering with the remaining ingredients.
6. Serve immediately and enjoy!

Prep time: 5 minutes.

Nutritional Information (Approximate):

• Calories: 300 kcal.

• Protein: 20g

• Fat: 8g

• Carbohydrate: 40g

• Fibre: 6g

• Sugars: 24g

42. Coconut Chia Seed Pudding:

Ingredients:

• 1/4 cup chia seeds.

• 1 cup coconut milk

• 1/2 teaspoon vanilla extract

• 1 tablespoon maple syrup, shredded coconut, and fresh berries for topping.

Instructions:

1. In a dish, combine the chia seeds, coconut milk, vanilla essence, and maple syrup.

2. Stir thoroughly and refrigerate for at least 2 hours or overnight.

3. Before serving, whisk the custard again to achieve a smooth texture.

4. Garnish with shredded coconut and fresh berries.

5. Enjoy your coconut chia seed pudding!

Prep time: 5 minutes (plus chilling time)
Nutritional Information (Approximate):
• Calories: 220 kcal.
• Protein: 4g
• Fat: 14g
• Carbohydrate: 20g
• Fibre: 8g
• Sugars: 10g

43. Baked Apples with Cinnamon and Walnuts:

Ingredients:
• 2 apples, cored and halved
• 2 tablespoons of chopped walnuts
• 1 tablespoon of honey or maple syrup.
• One teaspoon of cinnamon.
• One tablespoon of heated coconut oil.

Instructions:
1. Preheat your oven to 375°F (190°C).

2. In a small dish, combine the chopped walnuts, honey or maple syrup, and cinnamon.

3. Transfer the apple halves to a baking tray.

4. Fill the cored center of each apple half with walnut mixture.

5. Drizzle melted coconut oil over the filled apples.

6. Bake for 20-25 minutes, or until the apples are soft.

7. Remove from the oven and allow to cool slightly before serving.

Prep time: 10 minutes.
Cooking Time: 20-25 minutes.

Nutritional Information (Approximate):
• Calories: 200 kcal.
• Protein: 2g
• Fat: 12g
• carbs: 24g
• Fibre: 5g
• Sugars: 18g

44. Almond Butter Banana Bites:

Ingredients:
• Two peeled and sliced bananas.

• Two tablespoons of almond butter.
• Optional toppings include chia seeds or crumbled nuts.

Instructions:

1. Spread almond butter onto banana slices.
2. If preferred, add chia seeds or smashed nuts on top.
3. Place on a dish and serve immediately.

Prep time: 5 minutes.
Nutritional Information (Approximate):
• Calories: 180 kcal.
• Protein: 3g
• Fat: 10g
• Carbohydrate: 23g
• Fibre: 4g
• Sugars: 12g

45. Avocado Chocolate Mousse.

Ingredients:

• 2 ripe avocados
• 1/4 cup chocolate powder
• 1/4 cup maple syrup (or honey)
• 1 teaspoon vanilla extract

- 1 pinch salt
- (Optional), fresh berries for topping

Instructions:

1. Scoop avocado flesh into a blender or food processor.
2. Combine the cocoa powder, maple syrup or honey, vanilla essence, and a sprinkle of salt.
3. Blend until smooth and creamy.
4. Refrigerate the chocolate mousse for a minimum of 30 minutes.
5. Garnish with fresh berries if preferred.

Prep time: 10 minutes.
Chill time: 30 minutes

Nutritional Information (Approximate):
- Calories: 250 kcal.
- Protein: 4g
- Fat: 18g
- Carbohydrate: 27g
- Fibre: 8g
- Sugars: 15g

46. Greek Yoghurt and Honey Frozen Berry Popsicles.

Ingredients:
• 1 cup Greek yogurt
• 1 cup mixed berries (blueberries, strawberries, raspberries)
• 2 tablespoons honey
• Popsicle molds or sticks

Instructions:
1. In a bowl, blend Greek yogurt and honey.
2. Place a layer of the yogurt mixture in each popsicle mold.
3. Arrange a layer of mixed berries.
4. Continue adding layers until the molds are full, then top with a layer of yogurt.
5. Insert the popsicle sticks and freeze for at least 4 hours, or until completely firm.
6. After freezing, put the molds under warm water to remove the popsicles.

Prep time: 10 minutes.
Freeze time: four hours.

Nutritional Information (Approximate):

- Calories: 100 kcal.
- Protein: 6g
- Fat: 2g
- carbs: 18g
- Fibre: 2g
- Sugars: 15g

47. Quinoa and Almond Flour Brownies:

Ingredients:
- 1 cup cooked and cooled quinoa
- 1/2 cup almond flour
- 1/2 cup chocolate powder
- 1/2 cup maple syrup
- 1/4 cup melted coconut oil.
- 2 eggs
- 1 teaspoon vanilla essence
- 1/2 teaspoon baking powder.
- A pinch of salt.
- 1/2 cup dark chocolate chips.

Instructions:

1. Preheat the oven to 350°F/175°C and oil a brownie pan.

2. In a mixing dish, combine the quinoa, almond flour, cocoa powder, maple syrup, melted coconut oil, eggs, vanilla extract, baking powder, and a sprinkling of salt.

3. Add the dark chocolate chips.

4. Transfer the batter to the prepared pan and distribute it evenly.

5. Bake for 25-30 minutes, or until a toothpick comes out with moist crumbs.

6. Let the brownies cool before cutting them into squares.

Prep time: 15 minutes.
Cooking Time: 25-30 minutes.

Nutritional Information (Approximate):
• Calories: 150 kcal.
• Protein: 4g
• Fat: 9g
• Carbohydrate: 16g
• Fibre: 2g
• Sugars: 9g

48. Turmeric Golden Milk Ice Cream.

Ingredients:

• 2 cans (28 oz) full-fat coconut milk, chilled.

•1/2 cup maple syrup

• 1 teaspoon powdered turmeric

• 1/2 teaspoon ground cinnamon

• 1/4 teaspoon ground ginger

• One teaspoon vanilla extract

• A pinch of black pepper (improves turmeric absorption)

Instructions:

1. In a blender, mix cooled coconut milk, maple syrup, turmeric, cinnamon, ginger, vanilla essence, and black pepper.

2. Blend until smooth.

3. Pour the mixture into an ice cream machine and churn according to the manufacturer's directions.

4. Place the churned ice cream in a container and freeze for at least 4 hours, or until solid.

5. Scoop and serve, perhaps sprinkled with a pinch of turmeric.

Prep time: 15 minutes.

Churn Time: 20-30 minutes.
Freeze time: four hours.

Nutritional Information (Approximate):
• Calories: 200 kcal per serving (6 portions)
• Protein: 2g
• Fat: 15g
• Carbohydrate: 20g
• Fibre: 1g.
• Sugars: 15g

49. Pumpkin Spice Energy Balls.

Ingredients:
• 1 cup rolled oats
• 1/2 cup pumpkin puree
• 1/4 cup almond butter
• 1/4 cup honey or maple syrup
• 1 teaspoon Pumpkin Spice Blend
• 1/2 cup shredded coconut (to roll)

Instructions:
1. In a mixing bowl, combine the rolled oats, pumpkin puree, almond butter, honey or maple syrup, and pumpkin spice.

2. Mix well until a thick, sticky dough forms.

3. Refrigerate the dough for 30 minutes to make it simpler to work with.

4. Roll tiny bits of dough into bite•sized balls.

5. Roll each ball in crushed coconut to coat.

6. Put the energy balls on a dish and chill for at least an hour before serving.

Prep time: 15 minutes.
Chill Time: One Hour

Nutritional Information (Approximate):
• Calories: 90 kcal per energy ball (makes approximately 12 balls).
• Protein: 2g
• Fat: 5g
• carbs: 10g
• Fibre: 2g
• Sugars: 4g

50. Berry-Nut Yoghurt Bark:

Ingredients:
• 2 cups of Greek yogurt

- One cup of berry mixture (strawberries, raspberries, and blueberries).
- 1/4 cup chopped nuts (almonds and walnuts)
- Two tablespoons of honey or maple syrup.

Instructions:

1. Use parchment paper to line a baking sheet.
2. Spread the Greek yogurt evenly on the parchment paper.
3. Arrange the mixed berries and chopped almonds over top.
4. Drizzle honey or maple syrup over the yogurt.
5. Freeze for at least 4 hours, or until the bark solidifies.
6. After freezing, split the bark into smaller pieces.

Prep time: 10 minutes.
Freeze time: four hours.
Nutritional Information (Approximate):

- Calories: 120 kcal per serving (makes approximately 6 servings).
- Protein: 6g
- Fat: 5g
- Carbohydrate: 15g
- Fibre: 2g
- Sugars: 10g

Smoothies

51. Berry Bliss Smoothie:

Ingredients:
- 1 cup of mixed berries (strawberries, blueberries, raspberries)
- 1/2 banana
- Half cup Greek yogurt
- One-half cup almond milk
- One spoonful of chia seeds
- Ice cubes (Optional)

Instructions:
1. In a blender, combine the mixed berries, banana, Greek yogurt, almond milk, and chia seeds.
2. Blend until smooth.
3. If desired, add more ice cubes and combine again.
4. Pour into a glass and drink your Berry Bliss Smoothie!

Prep time: 5 minutes.
Nutritional Information (Approximate):
- Calories: 250 kcal.

- Protein: 12g
- Fat: 8g
- Carbohydrate: 35g
- Fibre: 8g
- Sugars: 20g

52. Green Goddess Hormone Balancer:

Ingredients:
- 1 cup kale leaves with stems removed
- 1/2 cucumber, peeled and sliced.
- One-half avocado
- 1/2 cup pineapple chunks
- One spoonful of flaxseeds
- One cup of coconut water.

Instructions:

1. In a blender, mix the kale leaves, cucumber, avocado, pineapple pieces, flaxseeds, and coconut water.

2. Blend until smooth.

3. Pour into a glass and enjoy the Green Goddess Hormone Balancer!

Prep time: 7 minutes.

Nutritional Information (Approximate):

- Calories: 220 kcal.

- Protein: 5g

- Fat: 14g

- Carbohydrate: 25g

- Fibre: 8g

- Sugars: 12g

53. Tropical Turmeric Smoothie.

Ingredients:

- 1 cup of mango chunks

- 1/2 banana

- Half cup Greek yogurt

- One-half teaspoon of turmeric powder

- 1 tablespoon honey

- 1/2 cup coconut milk.

Instructions:

1. In a blender, mix the mango chunks, banana, Greek yogurt, turmeric powder, honey, and coconut milk.

2. Blend until smooth.

3. Pour into a glass, and enjoy your Tropical Turmeric Smoothie!

Prep time: 5 minutes.
Nutritional Information (Approximate):
• Calories: 280 kcal.
• Protein: 9g
• Fat: 8g
• Carbohydrate: 45g
• Fibre: 5g
• Sugars: 35g

54. Chocolate Almond Joy Smoothie.

Ingredients:
• 1 cup almond milk
• 1/2 banana.
• 2 tablespoons almond butter
• 1 tablespoon cocoa powder.
• One tablespoon of shredded coconut.
• Ice cubes (Optional)

Instructions:

1. In a blender, mix almond milk, banana, almond butter, chocolate powder, and shredded coconut.

2. Blend until smooth.

3. If desired, add more ice cubes and combine again.

4. Pour into a glass and enjoy the Chocolate Almond Joy Smoothie!

Prep time: 5 minutes.
Nutritional Information (Approximate):
• Calories: 300 kcal.
• Protein: 8g
• Fat: 20g
• Carbohydrate: 25g
• Fibre: 6g
• Sugars: 15g

55. Hormone Harmony Berry Blend.

Ingredients:
• 1 cup mixed berries (blueberries, strawberries, raspberries)
• 1/2 cup Greek yogurt.
• One-half cup almond milk
• One spoonful of hemp seeds
• One spoonful of honey.
• Ice cubes (Optional)

Instructions:

1. In a blender, combine the mixed berries, Greek yogurt, almond milk, hemp seeds, and honey.
2. Blend until smooth.
3. If desired, add more ice cubes and combine again.
4. Pour into a glass and enjoy the Hormone Harmony Berry Blend!

Prep time: 5 minutes.
Nutritional Information (Approximate):
• Calories: 240 kcal.
• Protein: 10g
• Fat: 8g
• Carbohydrate: 35g
• Fibre: 6g
• Sugars: 22g

56. Mango Avocado Hormonal Booster:

Ingredients:
• 1 cup mango chunks.
• One-half avocado
• 1/2 cup coconut water
• 1 tablespoon chia seeds.

• One tablespoon of lime juice.
• Ice cubes (Optional)

Instructions:

1. In a blender, mix mango chunks, avocado, coconut water, chia seeds, and lime juice.
2. Blend until smooth.
3. If desired, add more ice cubes and combine again.
4. Pour into a glass and enjoy the Mango Avocado Hormone Booster!

Prep time: 5 minutes.
Nutritional Information (Approximate):
• Calories: 220 kcal.
• Protein: 5g
• Fat: 12g
• Carbohydrate: 30g
• Fibre: 8g
• Sugars: 20g

57. Spinach and Pineapple Power Smoothie.

Ingredients:
• 1 cup fresh spinach leaves

- 1/2 cup pineapple chunks.
- One-half banana
- 1/2 cup coconut milk
- One spoonful of chia seeds
- Ice cubes (Optional)

Instructions:

1. In a blender, mix the spinach leaves, pineapple pieces, banana, coconut milk, and chia seeds.
2. Blend until smooth.
3. If desired, add more ice cubes and combine again.
4. Pour into a glass and enjoy the Spinach and Pineapple Power Smoothie!

Prep time: 5 minutes.

Nutritional Information (Approximate):
- Calories: 180 kcal.
- Protein: 5g
- Fat: 8g
- Carbohydrate: 25g
- Fibre: 6g
- Sugars: 15g

58. Cinnamon Banana Nut Smoothie.

Ingredients:
- 1 cup almond milk
- 1/2 banana.
- 2 tablespoons almond butter
- 1/2 teaspoon ground cinnamon.
- One spoonful of flaxseeds
- Ice cubes (Optional)

Instructions:
1. In a blender, mix almond milk, banana, almond butter, ground cinnamon, and flax seeds.
2. Blend until smooth.
3. If desired, add more ice cubes and combine again.
4. Pour into a glass and enjoy the Cinnamon Banana Nut Smoothie!

Prep time: 5 minutes.
Nutritional Information (Approximate):
- Calories: 250 kcal.
- Protein: 8g
- Fat: 18g
- Carbohydrate: 20g
- Fibre: 6g

• Sugars: 10g

59. Hormone-Balancing Blueberry Bliss:

Ingredients:
• 1 cup blueberries, fresh or frozen.
• Half cup Greek yogurt
• One-half cup almond milk
• 1 tablespoon chia seeds
• 1 tablespoon honey
• Ice cubes (Optional).

Instructions:
1. In a blender, mix the blueberries, Greek yogurt, almond milk, chia seeds, and honey.
2. Blend until smooth.
3. If desired, add more ice cubes and combine again.
4. Pour into a glass and sip your Hormone Balancing Blueberry Bliss.

Prep time: 5 minutes.
Nutritional Information (Approximate):
• Calories: 230 kcal.
• Protein: 10g

- Fat: 8g
- Carbohydrate: 35g
- Fibre: 7g
- Sugars: 22g

60. Raspberry Coconut Elixir Smoothie.

Ingredients:

- 1 cup raspberries, fresh or frozen.
- 1/2 cup coconut milk
- One-half banana
- 1 tablespoon chia seeds
- 1 tablespoon shredded coconut.
- Ice cubes (Optional)

Instructions:

1. In a blender, mix raspberries, coconut milk, banana, chia seeds, and shredded coconut.
2. Blend until smooth.
3. If desired, add more ice cubes and combine again.
4. Pour into a glass and sip your Raspberry Coconut Elixir Smoothie!

Prep time: 5 minutes.

Nutritional Information (Approximate):

• Calories: 220 kcal.
• Protein: 5g
• Fat: 12g
• Carbohydrate: 30g
• Fibre: 8g
• Sugars: 18g

Chapter 5

Lifestyle Tips for Hormonal Health

Maintaining hormonal balance is more than just eating right; it requires a comprehensive strategy that takes into account many different aspects of life. In this chapter, we will look at three key aspects: **exercise, sleep, and stress management**, and how they all contribute to hormonal health. We'll also share practical strategies for incorporating these behaviors into your everyday routine.

The Impact of Exercise on Hormonal Balance

Exercise is essential for hormonal health since it influences the generation and regulation of important hormones in the body. Regular physical exercise can improve insulin sensitivity, decrease inflammation, and increase the release of endorphins, or feel-good chemicals. These components all contribute to hormonal balance.

To include exercise into your routine, aim for at least 150 minutes of moderate-intensity aerobic activity every week.

• Include strength training workouts at least twice a week to help maintain muscular health.

• Participate in activities you like, such as dance, hiking, or yoga, to make fitness a permanent part of your routine.

Prioritising Quality Sleep

The relevance of quality sleep in hormonal health cannot be emphasized. During sleep, the body goes through important activities including hormone control, cellular repair, and memory consolidation. Disrupting this cycle by persistently receiving little sleep can cause hormonal imbalances that affect mood, appetite, and stress levels.

To enhance sleep hygiene:

- Stick to a consistent sleep routine, going to bed and getting up at the same time every day.

- Establish a relaxing nighttime routine, such as reading or using relaxation techniques.

- Make sure your sleep environment is pleasant, dark, and silent.

Stress-Management Techniques

Chronic stress can destabilize hormonal equilibrium by stimulating cortisol release and altering other hormonal pathways. Integrating stress management tactics into your daily routine is critical for your general well-being.

To effectively manage stress, use mindfulness meditation or deep breathing techniques regularly.

- Participating in activities that provide delight and relaxation, such as spending time in nature, listening to music, or pursuing hobbies.

- Establishing realistic goals and boundaries to avoid undue stress from work or personal responsibilities.

Practical Tips for Developing Healthy Habits

1. Create a Balanced Exercise program: Adjust your program to fit your interests and lifestyle. If you just have a limited amount of time, high•intensity interval training (HIIT) can provide shorter but more effective exercises. Include friends or family to make exercise more fun.

2. Create a Sleep-Conducive Environment: Make your bedroom a haven for relaxation. For the best sleep, invest in a comfortable mattress and pillows, turn off electronic gadgets before bedtime, and adjust the room temperature.

3. Integrate Relaxation Techniques into Your Day: During breaks or stressful situations, engage in stress-relieving activities. Discover what works for you, whether it's a little meditation, a short stroll, or deep breathing exercises.

4. Prioritise Self-Care: Understand the significance of self-care in hormonal wellness.

Schedule time for things that offer you joy and relaxation, such as reading, bathing, or pursuing a hobby.

5. Listen to Your Body: Pay attention to the cues your body sends. If you're tired, take some time to relax. If you are experiencing excessive amounts of stress, consider altering your schedule or adopting additional relaxation practices.

To summarise, establishing hormonal balance is a complicated path that goes beyond food decisions. By embracing regular exercise, prioritizing great sleep, and successfully managing stress, you empower yourself to build a lifestyle that is in sync with your hormonal balance. Remember that little, persistent improvements can result in huge long-term advantages to your overall health and vigor.

Chapter 6

Personal Stories/Testimonials

Real-life experiences and testimonies about hormonal balance are compelling tales that appeal to those looking for a way to live a healthier lifestyle. In this chapter, we delve into personal experiences that not only emphasize the obstacles that women encounter while managing hormone imbalances but also celebrate the transformational journeys and accomplishments that result from determined efforts and the application of hormonal balance practices and recipes.

Personal Experiences with Hormonal Balance

Many women struggle with hormone changes, which cause a variety of symptoms and have an influence on their everyday lives. Sarah, a 45 year old professional, describes her effort to regain balance.

Sarah experienced prolonged exhaustion, mood swings, and irregular periods, all signs of hormonal imbalance. Frustrated with traditional therapies, she opted to take a more holistic approach, integrating nutritional food and lifestyle adjustments. Sarah's energy levels and mood improved gradually as she adopted a hormone-balancing diet, exercised regularly, and prioritized excellent sleep. Her example proves that with dedication and personalized treatment, it is possible to overcome hormonal issues and reclaim energy.

Transformational Journeys and Success Stories

Aside from the challenges, there are amazing success stories that demonstrate the transformational power of adopting hormonal balancing methods. Emma, a 50-year-old mother of two, discovered the powerful effects of diet on hormonal health.

Emma struggled with menopausal symptoms such as hot flashes and sleep disturbances. Unwilling to accept these as unavoidable, she sought advice and learned the function of certain nutrients in reducing menopausal symptoms. Emma added hormone-friendly meals to her diet, focusing on components like flaxseeds, omega-3-rich seafood, and antioxidant-rich fruits. With time, she noticed a significant reduction in hot flashes and felt more energized.

These personal tales highlight the diversity of women's hormonal balance experiences and the importance of personalized approaches to well-being. The testimonials show that adopting a holistic lifestyle, which includes a mindful diet and self-care routines, may result in good hormonal changes.

Impact of Hormonal Balance Practices

These stories highlight not just physical changes, but also the emotional and psychological empowerment that comes with hormonal balance. Women like Sarah and Emma demonstrate the power of resilience and rebirth when equipped with the information and resources to correct hormonal imbalances.

Empowering Others with Shared Experiences

Personal experiences and testimonials provide a sense of belonging and solidarity, informing women that they are not alone in their problems. They act as beacons of hope, inspiring others to begin their paths toward hormonal balance. The many routes these women have chosen remind us that there is no one-size-fits-all answer; rather, it is about determining what works best for each individual's well-being.

As we continue to investigate the many facets of hormonal health, these human tales serve as beacons of inspiration, demonstrating the transformational power of balanced nutrition, lifestyle choices, and self-care practices.

Conclusion

As we wrap off this exploration of hormonal balance for women over 40, it's critical to reflect on the important findings, empower women to prioritize their hormonal health, and give tools for ongoing learning and support.

Summary of Key Takeaways

Throughout this book, we've looked at the complex interplay of hormones in women over 40, as well as the tremendous effects that balanced nutrition, lifestyle choices, and recipes may have on hormonal health. Key lessons include understanding the relevance of hormonal balance, acknowledging the changes that occur at this period of life, and embracing a holistic approach that encompasses diet, exercise, sleep, and stress management.

We've looked at the importance of important nutrients and hormone-friendly components, as well as presented a multitude of recipes to help with hormonal balance. From breakfast to supper, snacks, and desserts, each cuisine exemplifies the delightful options that are consistent with hormonal health concepts.

Empowering Women to Prioritise Their Hormonal Health

This journey is about empowering women to prioritize their hormonal health. Recognizing the diversity of individual experiences, we've emphasized the need for tailored treatments, mindful diets, and self-care activities. The personal tales and testimonies featured in this book serve as beacons of hope, indicating that transformative journeys are possible.

Empowerment also comes from recognizing that hormonal health is a dynamic and ongoing process. It's about making educated decisions, developing a healthy relationship with one's body, and enjoying the path of self-discovery that hormonal balance implies.

Resources for Continuous Learning and Support

For people who want to understand more about hormonal health, there are several resources available to help them. Books, internet networks, and health specialists with expertise in hormonal balancing are all excellent resources. Staying educated and engaged enables women to manage their pathways with knowledge and confidence.

As a partner on this journey, I hope the thoughts, recipes, and anecdotes in this book have inspired you to feel empowered and curious. Hormonal balance is a journey, not a destination, and every woman can define her own story.

Finally, let this be an invitation to celebrate women's resilience, the transformational power of balanced living, and the exciting possibilities that come with prioritizing hormonal health. Here's to enjoying the journey, savoring nutritious food, and seeing a future in which women over 40 flourish with vigor, knowledge, and radiant health.

Appendix

In the quest for hormonal health, a thorough awareness of terminology and access to extra resources may be quite beneficial. This appendix supplements the knowledge offered in the book by providing a glossary of words and a curated list of additional reading and resources.

Glossary Terms

1. Hormones: Chemical messengers generated by glands in the endocrine system to control numerous physiological activities.

2. Oestrogen: The primary female sex hormone that controls the development and function of the female reproductive system.

3. Progesterone: A hormone that helps regulate the menstrual cycle and preserve pregnancy.

4. Insulin: A hormone that controls blood sugar levels by promoting glucose absorption into cells.

5. Cortisol: A stress hormone that regulates the body's fight-or-flight response.

6. Thyroid hormones (T3 and T4): regulate metabolism and energy generation.

7. Endocrine System: A network of glands that produces and secretes hormones into the circulation.

8. Perimenopause: The phase before menopause, marked by hormonal irregularities.

9. Menopause: The cessation of menstruation, which signals the end of the reproductive years.

10. Insulin resistance: A condition in which cells do not respond to insulin, resulting in high blood sugar levels.

11. Endorphins: are neurotransmitters that work as natural pain relievers and mood enhancers.

12. Omega-3 Fatty Acids: Essential fats with anti-inflammatory characteristics, necessary for hormonal balance.

13. Phytoestrogens: Plant chemicals that have estrogen-like actions in the body.

14. Adaptogens: Herbs that can help the body cope with stress and promote equilibrium.

15. Macronutrients: Nutrients that are required in significant quantities for normal body processes, such as carbs, proteins, and lipids.

16. Micronutrients: These are essential vitamins and minerals that must be consumed in small amounts for optimal health.

Suggested Readings and Resources

1. "The Wisdom of Menopause" by Christiane Northrup, M.D.: is an interesting book that explores the physical and emotional aspects of menopause.

2. "WomanCode" by Alisa Vitti: A book that investigates the relationship between hormonal health and the menstrual cycle.

3. "The Hormone Cure" by Dr. Sara Gottfried: provides a comprehensive approach to hormone balance via nutrition, lifestyle, and supplements.

4. "In the Flo" by Alisa Vitti: provides a complete guide to understanding and optimizing the menstrual cycle for hormonal wellness.

5. Websites: include Hormone Health Network (www.hormone.org), Women in Balance Institute (www.womeninbalance.org), and Endocrine Society (www.endocrine.org).

6. Online Communities: Joining online groups such as Reddit or health forums can offer support and insights from those going through similar hormonal health experiences.

7. Nutritionist and Functional Medicine Practitioners: Consult expert nutritionists and functional medicine practitioners for personalized hormonal health advice and assistance.

Remember that education is a valuable tool on the path to hormonal balance. These tools give a framework for comprehension, although individual experiences may differ. As you continue your journey, may you find the direction and support you require to embrace hormonal health with confidence and vigor.

Bonus: 21-Days Hormonal Harmony Meal Plan

Note: Adjust portion sizes based on individual needs and dietary preferences. This meal plan incorporates a variety of hormone-balancing recipes to support women's health over 40.

Day 1:

Breakfast: Berry Chia Seed Pudding

Lunch: Salmon Quinoa Bowl

Dinner: Grilled Turkey Burgers with Sweet Potato Wedges

Snack: Nut Butter Apple Slices

Day 2:

Breakfast: Quinoa Breakfast Bowl

Lunch: Chickpea and Vegetable Stir-Fry

Dinner: Cauliflower and Chickpea Curry

Snack: Trail Mix with Nuts and Seeds

Day 3:

Breakfast: Oatmeal with Flaxseeds and Berries
Lunch: Sweet Potato and Lentil Curry
Dinner: Lemon Garlic Herb Chicken with Roasted Vegetables
Snack: Hummus with Veggie Sticks

Day 4:

Breakfast: Smoothie Bowl with Green Leafy Vegetables
Lunch: Mediterranean Chickpea Salad
Dinner: Mushroom and Spinach Chickpea Pasta
Snack: Greek Yogurt Parfait with Almonds and Berries

Day 5:

Breakfast: Avocado Toast with Smoked Salmon
Lunch: Quinoa and Vegetable Buddha Bowl
Dinner: Shrimp and Broccoli Stir-Fry
Snack: Cottage Cheese with Pineapple

Day 6:

Breakfast: Vegetable Omelette with Broccoli

Lunch: Kale and Chickpea Salad with Tahini Dressing
Dinner: Salmon and asparagus foil packages
Snack: Seaweed snacks:

Day 7:
Breakfast: Berry Chia Seed Pudding
Lunch: Sweet Potato and Lentil Curry
Dinner: Quinoa Stuffed Acorn Squash
Snack: Nut Butter Apple Slices

Day 8:
Breakfast: Muesli with Flaxseed and Berries
Lunch: Turkey and Avocado Wrap
Dinner: Eggplant and Chickpea Stir-Fry
Snack: Greek Yoghurt Parfait

Day 9:
Breakfast: Whole Grain Pancakes with Blueberries
Lunch: Quinoa and Vegetable Buddha Bowl
Dinner: Vegetarian Lentil and Sweet Potato Stew
Snack: Pumpkin Spice Energy Balls

Day 10:
Breakfast: Quinoa Breakfast Bowl
Lunch: Mediterranean Chickpea Salad
Dinner: Turkey and Quinoa Stuffed Peppers
Snack: Turmeric Roasted Nuts

Day 11:
Breakfast: Vegetable Omelette with Broccoli
Lunch: Chickpea and Vegetable Stir-Fry
Dinner: Cauliflower and Chickpea Curry
Snack: Trail Mix with Nuts and Seeds

Day 12:
Breakfast: Avocado Toast with Smoked Salmon
Lunch: Sweet Potato and Lentil Curry
Dinner: Salmon and Asparagus Foil Packets
Snack: Hummus with Veggie Sticks

Day 13:
Breakfast: Greek Yogurt Parfait with Almonds and Berries
Lunch: Turkey and Avocado Wrap
Dinner: Lemon Garlic Herb Chicken with Roasted Vegetables

Snack: Berry and Nut Yogurt Bark

Day 14:

Breakfast: Whole Grain Pancakes with Blueberries
Lunch: Mediterranean Chickpea Salad
Dinner: Vegetarian Lentil and Sweet Potato Stew
Snack: Chia Seed Pudding

Day 15:

Breakfast: Berry Chia Seed Pudding
Lunch: Salmon Quinoa Bowl
Dinner: Shrimp and Avocado Salad
Snack: Roasted Chickpeas

Day 16:

Breakfast: Vegetable Omelette with Broccoli
Lunch: Kale and Chickpea Salad with Tahini Dressing
Dinner: Salmon and asparagus foil packages
Snack: Seaweed snacks:

Day 17:

Breakfast: Oatmeal with Flaxseeds and Berries

Lunch: Grilled Chicken Salad with Berry Vinaigrette

Dinner: Mushroom and Spinach Chickpea Pasta

Snack: Berry and Nut Yogurt Bark

Day 18:

Breakfast: Quinoa Breakfast Bowl

Lunch: Vegetarian Quinoa Stuffed Bell Pepper

Dinner: Grilled Turkey Burgers with Sweet Potato Wedges

Snack: Hummus with Veggie Sticks

Day 19:

Breakfast: Smoothie Bowl with Green Leafy Vegetables

Lunch: Salmon Quinoa Bowl

Dinner: Lemon Garlic Herb Chicken with Roasted Vegetables

Snack: Yogurt and Berry Smoothie

Day 20:

Breakfast: Avocado Toast with Smoked Salmon
Lunch: Quinoa and Vegetable Buddha Bowl
Dinner: Eggplant and Chickpea Stir-Fry
Snack: Chia Seed Pudding

Day 21:

Breakfast: Tofu Scramble with Vegetables
Lunch: Salmon Quinoa Bowl
Dinner: Grilled Turkey Burgers with Sweet Potato Wedges
Snack: Nut Butter Apple Slices

This 21-day meal plan provides a diverse range of nutrient-dense recipes to support hormonal health. Feel free to customize it based on individual preferences, and consult with a healthcare professional or nutritionist if needed.

About the Author

Amber K. Padilla is an accomplished author known for her expertise in creating cookbooks that cater to specific dietary needs. With a passion for cooking and a commitment to helping others, she has become a trusted source of recipes and information for individuals seeking healthier lifestyle choices.

In her book titled "Hormonal Balance Recipes For Women Over 40," Amber delves into the world of hormonal health diets, providing a comprehensive guide for women struggling with hormones-related health issues. Through extensive kitchen research, she has developed a collection of delicious and nutritious recipes that are specifically designed to support hormonal health. From flavorful breakfast dishes to satisfying smoothies, her cookbook offers a variety of options to ensure that women on a hormone healthy diet can still enjoy a wide range of tasty meals.

Amber's dedication to helping those with specific health concerns extends beyond the realm of hormone diets. She has also authored other notable cookbooks, including the "Beginners Renal Diet Cookbook", "Cancer Diet Cookbook" and the "Juicing for Cancer Recipes Book." These books provide valuable resources for individuals looking to incorporate healthy, cancer-fighting foods into their daily diet. With a focus on nourishing the body and supporting overall well-being, Amber's recipes are thoughtfully crafted to provide both taste and nutrition.

Furthermore, Amber has also explored the world of plant-based cooking with her "Vegan Instant Pot Recipes Cookbook" and "Anti-Inflammatory Recipes Cookbook." These books offer a wide array of plant-based recipes that support leading a healthy lifestyle while also being delicious. Whether someone is following a vegan diet or looking to reduce inflammation in their body, Amber's cookbooks provide a wealth of culinary inspiration.

Amber K. Padilla's kitchen research and passion for cooking shine through in her various cookbooks. With her dedication to creating healthy and flavorful recipes, she has become a go-to resource for individuals seeking dietary guidance and inspiration.